'That bit of help'

The high value of low level preventative services for older people

Heather Clark, Sue Dyer and Jo Horwood

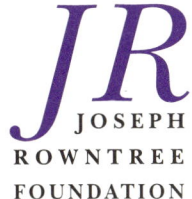

JR JOSEPH ROWNTREE FOUNDATION

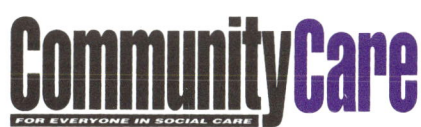

First published in Great Britain in 1998 by
The Policy Press
University of Bristol
Rodney Lodge
Grange Road
Clifton
Bristol BS8 4EA
UK
Telephone +44 (0)117 973 8797
Fax +44 (0)117 973 7308
E-mail tpp@bristol.ac.uk
http://www.bristol.ac.uk/Publications/TPP

© The Policy Press and the Joseph Rowntree Foundation, 1998
In association with the Joseph Rowntree Foundation.

ISBN 1 86134 118 0

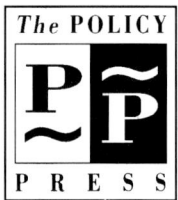

The *Community Care into Practice series* has been established by Community Care and
the Joseph Rowntree Foundation to make research available in the social care field to a
wide audience of managers and practitioners.

Community care is the leading magazine in the field of social care. It has supported this
report as part of its commitment to debate and the dissemination of information.

The report was written by **Heather Clark**, Senior Lecturer, School of Health Studies,
Chichester Institute of Higher Education; **Sue Dyer**, Principal Lecturer, Institute of
Nursing and Midwifery, University of Brighton and **Jo Horwood**, research assistant for
this project.

The Joseph Rowntree Foundation has supported this project as part of its programme
of research and innovative development projects, which it hopes will be of value to
policy makers and practitioners. The facts presented and views expressed in this
report, however, are those of the authors and not necessarily those of the Foundation.

Designed by Adkins Design.
Printed in Great Britain by Hobbs the Printers Ltd, Southampton.

Contents

Acknowledgements   4

Background to the report   5

Structure of the report   7

1   Introduction   9

2   The importance of domestic help   16

3   Moving between providers   32

4   The importance of safety and social participation   44

5   Themes and issues   51

6   Conclusions and implications   64

References   70

Acknowledgements

We would like to extend our thanks to all the practitioners and policy makers from the statutory and independent sectors for the help and support they have given us throughout the period of this study. We have also received tremendous support from and wish to thank Jackie Wilkins and Alison Jarvis of the Joseph Rowntree Foundation and the members of our advisory group: John Lansley, Shena Latto, Heléna Herklots, Frances Heywood, David Raw, Terry Stacey and Caroline Welch.

Most of all, we would like to thank the older people who took part in this study and who made us so welcome in their homes, sharing with us their experiences and perceptions. We are also grateful for the help of members of the pensioners' pressure group and the members of luncheon clubs and other social facilities who also shared their viewpoints with us.

Background to the report

There is a growing awareness among policy makers and practitioners of the value of preventative services in enabling older people to live independently within their own homes. There remains, though, a lack of national strategic planning and policy directives about preventative services. The want of a tool to measure their cost-effectiveness is also said to be an impediment to their development. This report argues that, important as it is to find ways of measuring the fiscal value of such services, the value older people give to preventative services cannot be ignored.

This report concentrates upon low level preventative services and the value older people give them. By 'value' we broadly mean the importance of such services to older people. Remaining in their own homes was the fundamental concern of the older participants in this study. This allowed them the exercise of choice and control that were central to their perceptions of independence. The older participants did not want to be looked after; they wanted to look after themselves as much as possible and the value they gave to low level preventative services was largely shaped by the extent to which such services did or would help them to do this.

At the same time, though, the older participants' definitions of independence were fluid, shifting in line with changing capacities and other circumstances. Help could be accepted with those tasks they could no longer manage without undermining the core concept of independence, so long as it did not impinge upon those areas that they could still manage for themselves. Our older participants consistently referred to the help they got, whether domestic or personal, as *help*, not care, illustrating that they perceived this as supporting them to look after themselves.

The report focuses upon a range of areas identified by older people as important to them: help with housework, gardening, house repairs and maintenance, security, laundry and opportunities for social participation. The consistency of the issues raised by our older participants was a remarkable feature of the research and, overwhelmingly, help with housework and domestic activities was stressed as vital to the maintenance of independence.

Many older people valued the relationship with the front-line provider as much as they did help with the task. The benefits derived from these relationships included feeling safe and cared about, while at the same time, making it easier for some to accept help. However, there were gender differences in the value accorded to help with housework and domestic tasks. While the older men tended towards a somewhat functional view of the value of domestic help, the older women perceived it in terms of skills and competencies. For the women in particular, the appearance of their homes was evidence of their ability to maintain acceptable standards and was linked to their public and private identities as competent adult members of their communities. The report therefore argues that such help is an important factor in ensuring the social inclusion of older people in general, and of older women in particular.

Structure of the report

Chapter 1 outlines the focus of the research and provides a short discussion of the policy context.

Chapter 2 examines the meanings of home and independence to older people and why help with housework is so important. It also questions the low value and low status accorded housework as a service and as an occupation. In contrast to the perceptions of some professionals who question the 'expert' status of front-line providers of domestic assistance, we present the perceptions of our older female participants. They viewed housework in terms of skills and competencies and accord it very high value in terms of the maintenance of their public and private identities and their ability to remain in their own homes.

Chapter 3 focuses upon a process whereby one local authority replaced its home help service with a voluntary sector provider and upon the perceptions and experiences of older people transferred between these providers. Particular attention is paid to the loss of affective relationships as a result of this transfer and the impact of that loss upon the older people's perceptions of the alternative provision.

Chapter 4 concentrates upon issues of safety and social participation. The value older people accord 'reputable' organisations such as Care and Repair for help within the home is discussed, as is the importance of safety devices. The fear of crime outside the home is recognised as contributing to the social isolation of older people and an anti-crime initiative which seeks to alleviate that fear by encouraging social participation is outlined.

Chapter 5 covers a range of themes and issues:

- the reluctance older people sometimes feel in asking for help – particular attention is paid to the difficulties in having to rely upon family support, which can be undermining of older people's feelings of independence, and the consequent value accorded to alternatives sources of help;

- how older people see services as *help* rather than *care* regardless of both their perceived level of need and the type of service they receive

– we argue that for older people what is important is that the services support them to care for themselves;

- professional boundaries and the issue of affective relationships are again raised – a case study is provided to highlight the dissonance between a professional and an older person's perception of independence;

- how older people shift their boundaries of independence in line with changes in their physical capacities and other circumstances – case studies are provided to illustrate this and a particular point is made of the inflexibility of some statutory services in supporting older people's desire to take care of themselves.

Chapter 6 comprises conclusions and implications of the research. In summary, there is a need for policy makers and practitioners to take account of:

- the meanings older people give to home and its importance to their public and private identities;

- the ways in which older people define independence and what they perceive as necessary to maintain it;

- the fluidity of older people's definitions of independence and the need for a flexible service response;

- the ways in which older people define assistance as help, not care, and the need to develop services which support their desire to look after themselves;

- the importance older people give to their relationships with front-line providers and the affective benefits they derive from these;

- the promotional and preventative value of services which enhance quality of life and encourage social engagement.

1

Introduction

Research focus

The starting point of the research underpinning this report concerned the value older people give to low level care and support services. Value is a contested concept but by it we mean the importance or worth older people themselves give to such services.

What constitutes 'low level' care and support services is open to a number of definitions and the central concerns of this report are to look at a range of such services and how older people view them. For many older people the term 'low level' probably has very little meaning. It is in effect a resource-led definition connected to the way in which older people's access to services is determined by eligibility criteria that have been developed as a means of rationing and thereby managing scarce resources. Within this context, the term low level is used to indicate low need, and therefore low in terms of both value and priority for resource allocation. This presents us with a problem of terminology: as this report makes clear the services described as 'low level' by professionals are those very services identified by older people as being of high value to them.

The areas consistently identified by our older participants as of high value were help with housework, gardening, house repairs and maintenance, security, laundry and opportunities for social participation. To understand the value of such services from the older person's viewpoint we have tried to broadly address the following questions:

- What matters to older people about these services?

- Does it matter who the provider is?

- Are these services about being cared for, or about being supported to self-care?

The concept of 'preventative'

The areas identified by our older participants fall under the broader remit of preventative services. In the main case study area in which this research was conducted the terms 'low level' and 'preventative' were used interchangeably, but with a discernible shift towards the latter. This may be seen to reflect a growing awareness of the value of preventative services in enabling older people to care for themselves and to maintain their homes such that need for more intensive, and indeed, more costly statutory support is held at bay. At the same time, it can reflect the shifting boundaries of local authority provision as services like help with housework are excluded from the core responsibilities of social services departments (SSDs) and in some areas may be then brought under the rubric of 'preventative'.

Increasingly SSDs have restricted their eligibility criteria, insofar as older people are concerned, to concentrate domiciliary services upon those perceived as posing a risk to themselves or others and/or those who without domiciliary support services would be unable to remain in their own homes. The needs for which SSDs currently accept statutory responsibility are primarily those where personal assistance is needed and older people who require help with solely domestic activities like housework may be excluded from statutory support. At the same time, however, some SSDs may define core services – including the provision of personal assistance[1] – as themselves preventative: the central problem here being that there is no agreed national definition of what comprises preventative services.

What preventative services are then is a vexed question. The short summary of proceedings from the joint seminar involving the Anchor Trust, the Association of Directors of Social Services (ADSS) and the Department of Health (DoH) (Anchor, 1996) on 'Preventative Services for Older People and Community Care' acknowledges the difficulty in defining preventative services but also states that there are two main groupings:

- 'services which prevent or delay the need for more costly intensive services such as nursing home care'[2] and

- 'services which promote the quality of life of older people and engagement with the community'.

These, as the summary says, are not necessarily mutually exclusive. The first grouping would include services which provide high levels of personal assistance as well as lower levels of domestic help: the underlying definition being led by a concern to prevent or delay a progression to or towards the need for the more costly provision of residential care. As the fuller report to the seminar indicates, preventative services might be seen as a way of using one service to prevent or delay the need to use another (Wistow and Lewis, 1997).

The evidence of the persistence of the 'perverse incentive' to residential care (Audit Commission, 1997) adds weight to the argument for improving domiciliary services to enable older people to remain in their own homes if that is what they wish. Yet if the line of preventative services is drawn at the point of admission to residential care or costly care packages indicating high levels of need, it can leave lower levels of service input vulnerable to the pressures upon SSDs to target resources upon these areas. There is, then, a need to consider a range of preventative services, including low level and low cost, as part of an overall preventative strategy. The services identified in this report fall within what we might call low level preventative services.

It has also been pointed out to us by senior professionals that as some SSDs struggle to meet their statutory responsibilities, they may be unwilling or unable to divert resources to promote quality of life and social engagement as ends in themselves without clear evidence of cost-effectiveness. The lack of a tool to measure cost-effectiveness has indeed stood in the way of developing preventative services in general (Wistow and Lewis, 1997). Yet in distinguishing between the preventative and promotional aspects of such services and concentrating solely upon people with complex levels of need, sight can be lost of just how effective those services can be.

Services which help older people manage those areas of daily life which are central to their preferred life-styles and independence can also help maintain their motivation to retain their independence (Wenger, 1992; Wistow and Lewis, 1997). This, as this report will show, applies regardless of levels of functional impairment. Cost-effectiveness has increasingly been reconceptualised as 'best value' and it is important for statutory agencies not to lose sight of the older person's priorities. An emphasis upon 'making resources meet demand' can mean a focus upon the *tasks* for which statutory agencies take responsibility and this in turn can preclude a focus upon *people.*

'Quality of life' has been subject to wide-ranging discussion and has been shown to have numerous and variable facets according to the preferences and circumstances of individual older people (Hughes, 1990; Sinclair and Williams, 1990a; Tinker, 1996). Services cannot provide quality of life; they can, however, enhance it. There is, though, an overwhelming need, if such services are to be effective, to listen to what older people say is important to them. The value of low level preventative services includes helping older people to take care of themselves and maintain their public and private identities as competent adult members of their communities.

Engagement with the community implies social inclusion. The report to the seminar cited above recognises the promotion of social inclusion as an important aim and outcome of preventative services (Wistow and Lewis, 1997). Insofar as older people are concerned, it is often discussed within the context of anti-poverty strategies aimed at giving information about and assisting take-up of state benefits. Important as these are, the presentation of self to the world as a competent adult is also a crucial factor.

National policy context

The twin aims of the reforms to community care embodied in the 1990 NHS and Community Care Act were to enhance independence and to promote choice among service users. It is stated in the White Paper *Caring for people* (DoH, 1989) that the proposals therein "would stimulate public agencies to tailor services to individual's needs". The thrust of the reforms was to achieve a shift from institutional-based services to community-based services in order to enable people to live independently and with dignity in their own homes or in 'homely settings' for as long as possible.

The White Paper stressed that the "successful implementation of community care policy depends crucially on the availability of, and ease of access to, adequate and appropriate services in the community" (para 1.4). The further development of a mixed economy of welfare was seen as central to stimulating the development of a wide range of services which would ensure greater choice, increased flexibility and innovation, and greater cost-efficiency.

Caring for people recognised that many older people who needed help and support might never become service users in the sense of being assessed and care managed. Yet, other than to stress the importance of access to information about local and national facilities and of supporting informal carers, little attention is accorded in the White Paper as to how their needs might be catered for. Indeed, the emphasis on providing services "that concentrate on those with the greatest needs" (para 1.10) may be seen to preclude statutory support for people whose needs are perceived as low level. The accompanying Policy Guidance states that local authorities may wish to look to the independent sector for the development of services, such as domiciliary and day care, to encourage innovative ways of meeting need (para 1.15). Again, however, there is no direct mention of preventative services for people outside of the care management process. There is, in other words, a lack of policy directive in terms of preventative services.

This makes it possible to interpret the White Paper and Guidance document in such ways as to promote preventative services. At the same time, of course, the permissive nature of both documents also means that there is no such statutory obligation. This, together with financial constraints, has probably contributed to their uneven development at national level and their endangered status where they do exist.

It would, however, be erroneous to equate the threat to low level preventative services solely with the implementation of the community care reforms and the emphasis upon targeting. In reality, targeting began in the 1980s (Wistow, 1997). One major service involved was the home help domestic service which was removed from the direct provider remit of many SSDs. Driving this was the recognition of an increasing need to provide a service to people with personal assistance needs in order to maintain them in their own homes rather than residential care. The question then facing SSDs lay in whether to continue to provide a larger number of older people with domestic help or to shift provision to provide a more intensive home care service but to fewer people (Henwood, 1992; Sinclair and Williams, 1990b; SSI,

1987). As Henwood says, the home care service came to be seen "as a substitute for residential provision" (p 17) – quite different to its historical development as a cleaning service predominantly for older people. The vacuum this left in terms of provision of services for people who did not meet the new eligibility criteria was "symptomatic of a wider strategic vacuum" (Wistow, 1997, p 2) which, in the absence of a coherent national policy framework, has yet to be addressed.

There is, however, room for cautious optimism about some areas of policy direction since the new Labour government came to power. For example, there is increased awareness of the need for a national drive within health and social services to prevent unnecessary admissions to both hospital and residential care. The Audit Commission (1997) has recently highlighted the potential of preventative services in this context. The White Paper, *The new NHS* (DoH, 1997) has promised greater integration of services for people with continuing health and social care needs. The Health Action Zone (HAZ) initiative aims to achieve better partnerships and reduce health inequalities, and to take into account the government's pledge to deal with the problem of social exclusion (Boateng, 1997). The recent Green Paper, *Our healthier nation* (DoH, 1998) identifies 'social exclusion' and 'quality of life' as health issues, and stresses that social services have a role to play in "fostering better health" by supporting people's independence and dignity (para 2.29). It remains to be seen, however, whether the social exclusion of older people will become a priority and whether or not the various initiatives will contribute to the development of low level preventative services which are integral to their social inclusion.

Finally, the Anchor Trust, ADSS and DoH joint seminar on preventative services referred to above has also generated interest, resulting in a Task Group being set up to take forward a programme of action, supported by the Department of Health (DoH). There are indications that a number of local authorities are beginning to develop preventative services and strategies. There are positive indicators that a number of local authorities are beginning to develop preventative strategies and services and the Task Group has commissioned a national survey of these and those of other sectors, including the health sector, voluntary sector and community organisations. The task Group has also set up a newsletter as a mechanism to share good practice and information.

About the research

The research was conducted in three local authority areas in the south of England and our older participants were contacted through a range of statutory and voluntary agencies and through their own friendship networks. Although we derived some of our 'data' from discussions with groups of older people, the bulk comes from individual interviews conducted in the homes of our older participants. Fifty-one older people were interviewed in their own homes and one third of these were interviewed on two or three separate occasions so that we could incorporate the impact of changing circumstances on their perceptions and experiences, particularly where those changes involved shifts in service provision. We undertook in-depth and very loosely structured interviews which, with the permission of the participants, were tape-recorded and transcribed by the interviewer.

We also interviewed professionals from the statutory and independent sectors ranging from senior managerial positions through to front-line providers, and consulted with members of a local pensioners' pressure group. Although our analysis is led by what our older participants told us, we have balanced this with the views of the professional participants, the pensioners' group and by reference to local and national policy.

We have called the major area in which we conducted the research 'the city'. We also included a 'rural area' where we concentrated upon domiciliary services, and a 'conurbation' where a safe cities scheme was in operation. The city and the conurbation became new unitary authorities during the course of this research, while the 'rural area' became part of a continuing authority.

Finally, we concentrated upon social rather than primary health provision. In this we were driven by the priorities of our older participants.

2

The importance of domestic help

Staying at home
The meaning of home and independence

During the early stages of the research it became clear that the older participants' views on low level preventative services were inextricably linked to their perceptions of *independence* and *home*. We have taken these views and linkages to the heart of this report because living independently within their own homes was the foremost concern of the majority of our older participants; the value they accorded low level preventative services was largely shaped by the extent to which they facilitated this.

The physical dwelling is important to most people but home can take on added significance in older age particularly if, as is the case with many of our participants, difficulties in going out alone means that increasing amounts of time are spent there. Older people conduct the majority of their social lives in their homes: family and others visit and conversations are conducted with friends by telephone – sometimes their major way of maintaining contacts and, as such, a 'lifeline'. Home locates the individual within a neighbourhood and therefore carries with it a private and social identity (Willcocks et al, 1987).

Home has a range of meanings for the older person (Gurney and Means, 1993; Langan et al, 1996; Sixsmith, 1986). For the majority of our older participants, it was interwoven with that of independence. One woman defined home as where it is possible "to do what I want, you know, and when I want. And have all the family here when I want", and independence as "being in my own home, my own space. That I've still got a bit of control over me, over my own life – that's what's important to me."

Our older participants saw remaining in their own homes as marking the final boundary of their independence and both were defined in terms of exercising choice and control over 'what you do', 'when you do it' and 'with whom you do it'. The older participants talked about residential care as something to avoid for as long as possible, if not forever, and a clear distinction was made between being *at* home and being *in* a home. For many, being in a home meant just sitting in armchairs around the edge of a room looking at each other. It meant not being able to "potter about" or "make a cup of tea" and having to fit into "a regime" or "obey the regulations" dictated by the organisation rather than follow one's own volition.

> "I wouldn't want to go into a home because I can please myself about what I do. Well you lose your independence don't you? And I mean because you've got to conform to a routine haven't you? And it's all laid down".

One woman talked about visiting her brother in a nursing home. Noticing that he had very dry lips, she asked him if he would like a cup of tea. "'Yes' he said, 'but I can't have one 'till 3 o'clock'". As this woman pointed out, "well in your own home you can go and make your own".

The loss of choice and control – in other words the loss of independence – was also equated with surrendering to the care of others, to being 'looked after'.

> "The independence is living on my own really. I don't want to go into *care,* if you know what I mean. You know – going into care and being looked after and being told what to do...."

Our older participants' determination to remain in their own homes was sometimes shaped by how long they had lived there, the efforts they had put into making the house a home, and the associated memories of their lives:

> "I married when I was 19, and moved here when I was 20 so I've been here, what, over 60 years in this house, and I like it here."

> "Of course my husband did a lot, when we first came, we created it. When I say we created it, that's why I didn't want to move, you know? He made the fireplace, there was a kitchen range in here ... [laughs]. Yes, it doesn't seem possible does it?"

Others who had moved home in later life stated that they had done so because their previous homes presented them with specific difficulties. Mrs Reid had moved because her privately rented house was damp; Mrs Callaghan because "the house was getting too big for me"; Mrs Styles wanted to "do away with gardens and things like that"; and Mrs Simpson because her previous flat "had a lot of steps inside and outside". Other than an absence of discussion about memories, there was really no difference in the ways they described the importance of home as enabling the exercise of choice and control, and the retention of independence.

Our older participants did not equate independence as the polar opposite of depending on others. In fact, they quite often used both terms to describe their lives but it was clear that being able to manage and stay in their own homes comprised the core identity of self as independent. This core self could be supported by others who helped them to cope with the tasks they could no longer manage themselves. It was in this context that some used the term 'depend'. This was acceptable so long as it supported the core identity of independence and did not incur a shift from having to depend on others for help to a total identity of dependency.

Independence becomes then a fluid concept, the boundaries of which change in line with changing capacities, energy levels and the availability of support and other resources. 'Care' is equated with being 'looked after' which implies a loss of self-direction, choice and control: a loss of one's public and private identity as an independent, competent adult.

Keeping the house up

The physical environment of the home can provide challenges to older people wishing to stay there, yet being able to master that physical environment despite any frailty is both empowering and confidence-building – enhancing capacities to manage and to interact with the world outside (Wilcocks et al, 1987). It was clear from our interviews that there was also an added dimension of gender. For the older women who participated in the research, home was the sphere where their competence as adults was evidenced by their ability to maintain standards of housework such that they felt comfortable with the public image their homes presented. This related to their own levels of well-being in terms of how they perceived their home from inside, as well as their confidence in inviting people to come into their home.

Most of our older female participants linked keeping the house up with keeping themselves up. Public and private esteem were linked to the appearance of their home and importantly to their own perceptions about their ability to stay there:

> "Well you go down if you let the house go down, don't you? If you're not troubled about the house, you're not troubled about yourself are you? No you must keep over plimsoll line, dear, keep yourself up regardless." (Mrs George, 82 years)

The following case studies also serve to illustrate this theme.

Mrs Styles was in receipt of personal assistance. As she put it, she 'qualified' for housework by "qualifying for what they call personal care." It was clear that she most valued the help with the former. Mrs Styles said of the help she got with her housework: "by giving us that now, they're enabling us to stay in our own homes" and that means "they don't actually have to pay for us going into a home and please God I never do!" This statement, echoed by other participants, suggests that help with housework *prevents* admission to residential care.

Mrs Styles got help with strip washing and dressing on three mornings, amounting to one-and-a-half hours per week. Before the shift from home help to home care, she had received four hours per week with a much greater emphasis upon housework. The reduction in help with housework, together with her concerns about *who* she might get from home care led her to employ her ex-home help (Betty) in a private capacity:

> "Well actually Betty retired … and I was a bit perturbed because over the time when Betty's been either on holiday or sick or anything, you get reliefs come in and I mean I didn't know quite who I was going to get when Betty retired … so I said to Betty would she come and do my housework."
>
> At the same time, though, Mrs Styles did not want to lose her home care input "just in case":
>
> "I wanted to keep my foot in the door because I mean if at any time Betty goes on holiday or anything I shall want somebody to come in more often and, er, actually I've been extremely lucky with the two girls I've got, they're both lovely girls".
>
> Mrs Styles would not get more home care hours if she didn't have Betty because 'personal care' is the major focus of the service and housework is very much a secondary consideration.

Home care managers told us that there are clients who receive a specified 'slot' for housework each week but more usually the home carer fits a little bit of cleaning into the odd 10 minutes that may be left when the personal assistance tasks have been completed. In any case, cleaning is restricted to the main living areas, the kitchen, bathroom and toilet.

In the city area, home care managers advised us that the service had been reorganised during the late 1980s, with the major focus switching to providing personal assistance. However, changes had been incremental so some clients continued to receive a housework-based service (see Chapter 3 for further details). Despite transitional arrangements, a change in circumstances or an 'exit' from the service could lead to being 'excluded' from help with housework.

Mrs Jones, a widow in her 80s, lives in Part II accommodation in the city. About nine or ten years ago, she was in hospital with "a heart problem".

> "The doctors arranged home help and I had a home help for about two-and-a-half years. My home help went sick and they kept sending reliefs and I wasn't happy about it so I cancelled it. I saw my home help the day I cancelled it and she said 'you can't be without a home help, you've got to have them' but they wouldn't put me back on it so I went private".

Mrs Jones could not remember exactly what the home care manager had told her other than: "'you don't need us', or something." She felt that the switch from home help to home care indicated a lack of understanding of what was important: "Why is it that home care cannot do any housework because that is important as much as anything else isn't it – to someone who can't do housework?"

Like so many others, it was the *work* of housework rather than the *care* of personal care that counted:

> "They take the home help away and they give you a home care but that home care is not doing any work. They come to see if they can help you in any way body-wise or shopping so what happens to the work the home help used to do. That has been my query, you know. Because you can't really cope, I mean I've got to get someone in to do my work, I can't do it on account I have aïsthma and ... erm ... a little bit of heart problem that goes with it, so I have to depend on someone to do my floor work. I mean ... how can I put it? I can do dusting, anything that's eye level, but when it comes to anything high or pushing, I can't do it".

One of our participants could not get support in providing personal assistance to a relative when she needed it, nor support with housework once help with personal assistance was no longer necessary.

Mrs Callaghan is 80 and lives alone. Her husband was killed during the Second World War and she and her son went to live with her parents-in-law. As they aged, she became their primary care-giver, first for her father-in-law until his death, and then for her mother-in-law. As her mother-in-law became increasingly frail, Mrs Callaghan helped her with personal and domestic tasks: "I used to help her have a bath and dress and I did all the cooking and cleaning".

Mrs Callaghan provided this assistance alone until she was in her 70s. She then got home help to assist with housework but could not get help to bathe her mother-in-law: "No. When I wanted a nurse to help me bath her, that was something else they'd cut out of the services so we managed."

Eventually Mrs Callaghan could no longer manage to lift her mother-in-law and their GP persuaded them that she should go into residential care:

"The doctor said I couldn't go on. It was getting too difficult and I couldn't lift her. With my arthritis the doctor could see it was getting too much worry. They persuaded her to go in ... and she fought hard against it. I don't think she ever forgave me for putting her in a home but I couldn't cope with her any longer".

Mrs Callaghan informed 'social services', advising that she still wanted home help:

"... and they came back and said 'Mrs Callaghan, your home help is stopping, you're not entitled to home help now', because mother had gone. So I said, 'Well I need it, it's me that needs it, doing the work'. 'Oh well, we will assess you if you want, but you're not entitled to any home help'. So I think my son politely told them what to do...."

Mrs Callaghan expressed her feelings at the time:

"I felt flaming mad, I thought well it's me been doing all the work. She's just been sat here and done nothing, it's me that wants the home help. I know I'd got it with having her but when she'd gone, well...."

It would seem that Mrs Callaghan lost out at both points of the transition: when she needed help to bathe her mother-in-law, that was not available; now that she needs help with her housework, she is not eligible.

She has in fact employed the ex-home help's daughter: "I pay for that privately, it's nothing to do with them 'cos they said I wasn't entitled to it". As for so many of our female participants, the preventative value of housework was clear:

> "Thank goodness I can pay for the help I want because as I said rather than go in a home I would rather pay someone you know to come in and do more. That's what I would prefer, to live in my own home for as long as possible."

Like a number of our older participants in the city area, Mrs Styles, Mrs Jones and Mrs Callaghan had organised their own domestic help – their own preventative services. And as was the case with others, they did this through existing links with their ex-home helps/home carers. Mrs Styles was happy with the help she continued to receive from home care primarily because she liked the 'girls'. The others were extremely unhappy with the changes to the home care service because it meant the loss of a form of help which they saw as essential to enabling them to remain in their own homes.

In the rural area, similar themes were raised, although here home help was still available on a limited basis – limited in part by the costs incurred in travelling, and in part by recurrent cash crises in the wider local authority area.

Mrs Cox was a widow in her 90s. Help with her housework meant that she felt she could have visitors to her home: "I think you've got to feel it's reasonably presentable because I've never minded people dropping in ... but you feel that you want to be prepared don't you."

She also, however, knew other older people who couldn't get this help and was concerned that not only could she not get additional help but that what she currently got was under threat: "I think they're trying to knock it down now because they are so hard pushed for money. It's the money all the time."

This she saw as social services failing to understand the importance of housework to older people:

> "Well, they don't understand. Oh, I know there's lots of things they don't understand – they don't think housework is necessary, now can you understand that? I suppose you're just supposed to sit here and look at it. I can't understand that can you?"

For Mrs Cox, as with many other older women, how she felt about her physical surroundings and how confident she felt about inviting other people in were both distinct and related issues.

It seemed that for most of our older female participants, housework was closely linked with their self-esteem, well-being and public and private identity as competent adults. As a member of a pensioners' pressure group in the city put it:

> "The important thing about home help was that a person living on their own needs to present an image of home as sailing along as it used to be – it's very important to them to maintain the status quo in the environment in which they choose to live."

What matters to women

As we progressed with this research we formed the perception that housework was not regarded as a professional service and that those who undertook the task were not regarded as 'professionals' by others within the SSD. The low status accorded to housework as an occupation, as unskilled work, was further reflected in the low priority accorded to the service. One senior professional questioned the 'professional' status of both home helps and home carers on the basis that they sometimes crossed professional boundaries by forming extra-work relationships with their older clients. This, she said, precluded them from the status of 'expert'. In general, however, those involved in policy planning did not regard housework as an essential service because needing such help "is not life-threatening".

Our older female participants would take issue with these perceptions. Mrs Kennedy put it so:

> "It's all very well saying 'Oh well, it's only housework' – I know myself that when I came out of hospital, I couldn't do any housework. And the dust just builds up and builds up and there was no way that I ... I mean I was flat on my back on the settee for most of the time. And ... if you don't ... if you're not used to that sort of thing, it plays on your mind. And you think to yourself 'Ooh ...' – it's not only your own *body* that you're thinking of ... – you're thinking about all this dust building up, aren't you?"

Help with housework can be important to older people's mental health, assuaging the anxiety and loss of self-esteem that can come with the inability to keep the house clean. A lack of such help can also increase risk-taking and, as a consequence falls, as older people struggle to manage for themselves (House of Commons Health Committee, 1996).

Many of the women talked about their home carers as experts. This was stated in relation to the housework they performed. Mrs Ashton, like many other women used a discourse often reserved for nurses, stating that home carers are "marvellous – absolutely" and "not doing it for the money."

> "Yes. They're all very good – they do whatever they can in the hour and, you know, they just whip it quickly all round. They're really good – I was absolutely amazed. I'd heard that they weren't all that good, but they certainly are here, whatever they are anywhere else – they're *experts* and they look as though they like doing their work, you know ... they know the ropes absolutely and what needs doing."

The older women tended in general to perceive the tasks of housework more in terms of skills and competencies than did the men, who had a more functional view. For the women, too, the appearance of their homes was centrally linked to their perception of their public and private identity and some reported that their late husbands had helped them to retain this by helping with the housework.

The research indicated that women's relationship to the home is different to men's. Men and women's self-identity is constructed to varying extents upon gender socialisation and for older people, traditional gender roles whereby women take primary responsibility for domestic tasks, may be more pronounced than among younger generations. Today's older women probably had, as girls, a much more thorough apprenticeship in domesticity (Oakley, 1974) and the performance of domestic tasks is central to the self-identity of many older women (Arber and Ginn, 1991). However, there does not appear to be any recognition of this in national policy and guidance documents, nor does it appear to be given any attention in local policy planning. There seems to be a 'policy myopia' about gender, which is doubly surprising when one considers the predominance of women among both the older age groups and those older people experiencing functional impairment.

This is not to say that all SSD providers fail to recognise the particular importance of housework to women. One provider manager was concerned about the lack of policy directive in terms of targeting housework services for women and stated:

> "I mean if there's a statement made about those gender issues I would be delighted, it's not something that's talked about at all."

This provider manager was concerned that what she called her "army of women" – her home helps – "who go about their business and keep other women happy and keep their houses clean" were consistently undervalued by the rest of the service.

Net curtains: the meeting of the public and the private identity

In this research the problem of changing net curtains was the most mentioned single housework task. Perhaps this is not surprising given that 'nets' not only afford privacy indoors but also comprise both a private and public display of housework competence and respectability. Net curtains probably signified the meeting of the public and private more than any other single housework-related issue.

Mrs Butler, a widow of 93 living alone, was experiencing a number of difficulties. She found it difficult to get out of her chair, she had to pull herself upstairs by holding on to the banister and come down backwards, and she had recently fallen in her garden and had to crawl to her kitchen to pull herself up on the sink and oven. She was, however, more concerned about the problems she faced in changing her net curtains and the covers on her suite. A lodger used to help her but had now moved away "so I shall need help now 'cos I always change my curtains and put other covers on my suite". For Mrs Butler, having clean nets was an outward sign of respectability; having "mucky nets" was evidence that "they haven't troubled to wash them".

Mrs Smith, a widow aged 81, became tearful as she explained that her curtains "were filthy". Following a fall two weeks before our first meeting no housework had been done. She explained to the researcher during the second visit that the curtains "have never been that colour in my life" and that before her fall, they had been "religiously done". She used to, she said, "drag the steps upstairs", stepping from them onto a blanket box under the window to change her nets: "It took a time but I did it". As she aged, this became more difficult and after her fall she became afraid of damaging her back again.

Mrs Smith had been widowed for, as she put it, "four *long* years". She told us that when her husband was alive he had increasingly taken on some of the housework "to save me":

> "I mean it took a time after my husband died because we were like a team – we worked together. And I was completely lost when he went and when I used to do jobs that we used to do together and it was *hard* for me, I'd say 'Help me, help me to do it right'. And I'd *do* it rather than ask for help. But as I said, since I've turned 80, the body won't let you."

Mrs Smith became tearful each time she mentioned her husband; she missed him terribly and she kept his cap and his slippers in their old usual place. As the above quote indicates, she often spoke to him when she found something hard to manage. She was determined to maintain standards: "I can't let the place go".

Mrs Smith's situation highlights how loss of a partner in later life can exacerbate the impact of existing impairment in both tangible and intangible ways. It's like a "dripping tap" (Stevenson, 1989): thoughts go back to "when my husband was alive" and the grief and feeling of loneliness are inseparable from the reality of the difficulties now faced. While, as we have stated, home holds an extra dimension for women in terms of their self-identity, there is also the need for a public image "of home as sailing along as it used to be". Mrs Smith's husband had helped to maintain this. After his death Mrs Smith had coped with the task of changing the curtains in what might be regarded as a somewhat risky way. She now felt that the risk was too great and needed help. Yet there is no formal provision of help for such tasks – indeed, home carers and home assistants are not supposed to use steps or ladders during the course of their work in older people's homes because it is considered too risky. Who then is supposed to do it?

Our pensioners' pressure group members asked the same question and added:

> "The ageing process diminishes people enough – but in common with everyone, they don't want to lose self-respect; their own perceptions of themselves. People still try to do things like nets and end up having accidents, yet can't get paid help to do it."

Mrs George solved the problem by having the Care and Repair Handyperson service lower the curtain rails so that she could change her nets. For her the service was very important:

> "They're fantastic! I've got my list somewhere, I've written it all down. All the curtains so I can reach them. It's all right if you've got somebody in the house but I haven't so I've got to depend, and if I fall down here, nobody might see me for days".

Although Mrs George lives in her back room, she first had the rails in the front room lowered – that is to say, the ones facing the street. At the same time, her rationale for the work is safety – to be able to *safely* reach her curtains.

For others in our sample group, difficulties in changing their nets and dealing with other aspects of housework are a constant physical reminder of what they are no longer able to do:

> "You just don't think of yourself as old and it's only when you come up against something that you can't do, I can't get on steps now to get up to the shelf, that you realise."

Many experience problems with 'hoovering' as they can no longer push the vacuum cleaner. Lifting and carrying washing is too heavy for some, bending to clean floors or cookers is hard or impossible for many, and ironing can exhaust energy levels. Whenever we asked older people what they valued about the services they got, help with housework and household tasks was stated almost unanimously by the women as the priority. This was the case whether or not the older person was in receipt of personal assistance. Such help would or did enable them to cope and to remain in their own homes.

What matters to men

Men living alone did not display the same level of concern about the public image the house presented, nor did help with housework appear to be related to their sense of independence. Mr Pinter, for example, simply saw its value in giving him the "freedom" from worry about standards and stated very clearly that such help was unrelated to his sense of independence. In fact, we found that the men rarely talked about independence in any way that suggested it was under threat or indeed that it was an issue.

Some of the older men used a quite different language when discussing the help they received. Mr Lacey, a widower of 92, referred to his home carer as "the cleaner", while Mr Williams, in his late 90s, talked about the "the cooks". Neither man had done any cooking when their wives were alive and to some extent the tasks performed by their home carers replaced those done earlier by their wives:

> "The wife took more responsibility for the house, you know, cooking and all that. I was alright ... I didn't do anything in that line, I wasn't that way inclined."

Since his wife's death, Mr Williams has taken up his old love of dancing which he was able to pursue at a local 'blind club'. He could have attended this club several times a week but went only on the evening which is "given over to refreshments". He also attended a luncheon club once a week, which he enjoyed because he was "outnumbered by the womenfolk".

Mr Williams wanted to stay in his own home where he could "... carry on in my own sweet way". When asked about independence, however, Mr Williams talked more about "taking a walk". There was no discernible link between domestic tasks and his own sense of independence. What was clear though was the importance of food, as it was for Mr Lacey, "if I get a little help for a clean up and meals it's all I want". For the men, their own self-identity was far less tied to the home than that of the women.

For one man, however, the loss of his wife to a nursing home undermined the status of house as home: "This is no longer a home with my wife not here; it's just a house that shelters me from the elements."

Human relationships were important to Mr Andrews. He pointed out that "my home help is terribly important to me, for they're, as it were, social contacts, they're friends". In his own terms, he has his "basic needs" met: meals on wheels, a weekly bathing service, shopping and housework. His appreciation of these services was stated in rather less than aesthetic terms – he simply defined himself as "an untrained mere man" whose house is therefore "looked after by home help". His home help, however, takes him each week to see his wife, which is clearly very important to him as he gets "very sad with my wife not being here".

A particular dimension to the rather more functional value men accorded to help with domestic tasks is illustrated by one of our case studies in which the husband had assumed the role of care-giver for his wife.

Mr and Mrs Laws are 90 and 89 respectively. Their only relative, a niece, lives five hours drive away. Mrs Laws has Alzheimer's disease and her husband had been caring for her for at least two years. They had twice-daily home care for Mrs Laws' personal assistance needs, plus two separate hours per week for housework. Mr Laws had been reluctant to accept home care on the basis that "I thought, well ... it will take a bit of my independence away".

Mr Laws clearly found it difficult to accept help. He had very exacting standards and he really didn't believe the home carers, who he described as "that assortment of women that comes up here" could do the personal and domestic tasks as well as he could. Nevertheless, he did find that having help with some housework tasks – particularly ironing – allowed him to pursue his own hobbies. His wife, he said, "sometimes plays the devil" and spending time alone in his workshop "settles me down" and allowed him to "face coming back and dealing with everything".

Although Mr Laws felt that he could manage without the help, he was concerned that he might suddenly need it if his wife's condition deteriorated or he himself became incapacitated:

> "I'm afraid – she might fall next week. I'm afraid to say I can do without it and then needing it again next week – that's what I'm afraid of. Something could happen to me and if I've got these people coming in they'd probably see about it."

He was also concerned that it would take some time to re-enter the system:

> "Well I can't run around and get care all of a sudden ... You can't get it in a minute because they come up and interview you and goodness knows what and all that."

It can be seen from the above case study that, although Mr Laws had mixed views about the service received (he felt he could do it better), he did appreciate the back-up and the opportunity for space for himself. Unlike our female participants, however, there was no sense in which he or the other men linked their own identities to the help they received.

3
Moving between providers

From home help to home care: the process

During the 1980s, SSDs were faced with the problem of whether to continue to provide a larger number of people with domestic help or to switch to a more intensive home care service to fewer clients. Different SSDs reacted differently to the challenge. Some retained a home help service; others shifted to providing help with housework only for those clients in receipt of personal assistance. The city's response provides a case study in itself.

In the city there was an incremental withdrawal from the provision of a solely domestic help service. The precise history of that process is difficult to determine for a number of reasons, not least of which is that the city is a new unitary authority. Consequently, the policy directives concerning what core services should comprise, how services should be targeted and what resources should be made available came until recently from the 'mother' local authority. Furthermore, interpretation of these directives at local area level appears to have been far from uniform.

Nevertheless, it is clear that in the late 1980s the home care service itself was reviewed, and part of that review focused upon a disparity of provision across the then wider county. One outcome was that the city lost around 600 hours of home care provision as part of a policy of reallocation of hours. The city then moved towards the first of a two-stage process. The first stage comprised the decision *not to accept* any more new referrals for housework only. The second stage involved *withdrawing* the home care service from those older people who required only domestic help. According to one senior manager from the 'mother' authority, the shift to 'personal care' also resulted from the pressures to target "those most in need and make effective use of money". It marked "a reaffirmation of the fact that home help was moving away from preventative or low level services to ones of providing personal care".

An announcement in the local press that social services would no longer provide a home help service led, as it did in other areas of the county, to a groundswell of opposition by older people themselves and by agencies representing their interests. Through this, significant political pressures were brought to bear. In the meantime, a large voluntary organisation in the city set up a scheme which, rather like a dating agency, brought older people who wanted help with housework and shopping together with individuals, operating on a self-employed basis, who could offer such a service at an affordable rate. However, the demand began to outpace the voluntary organisation's resources, particularly the infrastructure costs.

The political pressure found major expression in the local planning group for older people, involving representatives from social services, health, housing, a range of carers groups, voluntary organisations, and pensioners' groups. At the same time, the new local government administration had committed itself to providing a domestic service for older people. However, the use of a relatively expensive and increasingly sophisticated home care service for cleaning was judged untenable and housework was to remain outside the 'core business' of social services. A lengthy policy process followed, the eventual outcome of which was that the local authority put out tenders for a housework service. This targeted the voluntary sector, in part because of the need for cost-affordability and in part because of the preferences of the local political administration.

The contract was awarded to the voluntary organisation's home assistance scheme, now renamed Help in the Home (HITH). The terms of the contract and funding arrangements between social services and the voluntary organisation are unusually prescriptive. The service is confined to older people who do not require personal assistance with a maximum of two hours per week help allowed. Charges are pre-set, including a reduced rate for older people in receipt of income support, as is the hourly rate of pay for the assistants. Originally assistants were paid only for the work they performed, although since September 1997 they are guaranteed four hours pay per week. Their hours are limited in order to avoid National Insurance liability, and they are not entitled to sick or holiday pay. This, then, is a flexible labour market made up of predominantly women. However, that very flexibility, as will be explained below, led in some instances to inflexibility of service provision.

With the setting up of HITH, social services began to withdraw home care from those older people who required help with only housework and shopping. The older people to be transferred were informed by letter six weeks before the withdrawal, although in general home carers seem to have delivered the 'news' to their clients. Some home carers were themselves unhappy with the shift towards personal care and the related changes to their contracts of employment. It seems that this, together with their relationships with individual older clients, may have exacerbated some older people's distress.

Those responsible within the city SSD for the shift readily admit with hindsight that it could have been handled better. While a relatively small number of older people were shifted from one service to another, the process could hardly be described as seamless. Attempts were made to ensure that there were no gaps in service provision, yet little acknowledgement was made of the disruption experienced by some older people in terms of the relationships developed between them and their home carers.

The outcome for older people: the loss of affective relationships

For some of our older participants, the transfer from home care to the independent sector, involving as it did the loss of valued relationships, initially impacted negatively upon their perceptions of the independent provider. That they were informed of the transfer by their home carers exacerbated their distress. The following case studies illustrate these points.

Mrs Kennedy is a widow in her 70s. She has osteoporosis and had home care for six years before she was transferred to HITH. Her views on the switch from home help to home care were expressed thus:

"I personally think it was one of the worst things that they did when they took the home help away from the council – from the social services, as they did. You know, if they'd had perhaps a two-tier system ... 'cos I had a lovely home help. It gets depressing if you can't do these things. It was wrong and that, you know, how it affected people mentally if they couldn't get the service – the help for doing their housework."

Mrs Kennedy told us that she had had the same "excellent" home help/home carer for many years:

> "You see I'd had Wendy for so long that, you know, you build up a relationship with people don't you? I mean, she was almost like a daughter to me, you know. And I always knew I could rely on her. I mean, I know they're not supposed to give out their home telephone number but I had hers and if ever ... whether it was her day for coming or not, you know – I could always phone her up and say 'Oh Wendy, I'm in trouble – can you pop in?'"

Mrs Kennedy also thought the process had been poorly managed:

> "I think it was so badly done as well. Because she had to tell me, she was the one that had to tell me that she was having to leave ... and she was, you know, quite upset about it as well."

It took some time for Mrs Kennedy to settle into the new service. She was very unhappy with her first assistant, finding both the quality of her work and her time-keeping poor. When, however, she left and was replaced by a woman who had previously been a home help, Mrs Kennedy was far happier. Her new assistant had left social services because she, according to Mrs Kennedy, "couldn't cope with personal care". Mrs Kennedy did tell us, however, that she was left with no help for three weeks between the two HITH assistants and remarked upon how the "dust built up and built up" during that period. She found this depressing.

Mrs Kennedy was also aware that her new home assistant was paid only for the hours actually worked, meaning that she didn't like to cancel her service if she wanted to do anything else:

> "I don't think personally that their conditions are very good. They don't get paid holidays. And if I say 'Oh I don't want you this week' – if you're working for the social services, you still get paid those hours but with (HITH) they don't get paid those hours. They only get paid for the hours that they *actually* work, you know. And I mean, they could be a person who relies on that money."

Mrs Kennedy was not the only older participant who experienced gaps in service provision:

Mrs Rutherford, a widow of 87, was distressed by the loss of the home carer who had been with her for 11 years. Mrs Rutherford has no immediate family and although she told us that she had "no friends", she did have "good neighbours" with whom she had a reciprocal relationship: they helped with shopping, she baked cakes for them and they all regularly met in her house for tea and cakes. It seemed Mrs Rutherford's neighbours provided practical rather than emotional support.

Her relationship with her ex-home carer had been very important to her and she described her several times as " like a little daughter to me". Again it was the home carer who broke the news of the service withdrawal. Mrs Rutherford said that at the time she felt "Rotten! I'd got so used to her you see". However, she did come to terms with the change and when we visited her again six months later she described her home assistant as "a very nice woman". However, this was the second assistant she had had; the first "broke everything she touched".

Although the current assistant was described as "excellent", she had not yet had the chance to develop the same sort of relationship she had enjoyed with her home carer since she had only been there for three weeks. However, Mrs Rutherford did say she was "very nice to talk to" which was important to her:

"Because you see, actually speaking, I'm the last one of my family – I haven't got anybody barring me two nieces and ... you see, they're getting on".

Mrs Rutherford was more than satisfied with the work done – "she does it lovely" – and talked of why the appearance of her home was so important to her:

"I've been told I'm too fussy but you can't be too fussy though. I like everything nice and clean. That's the only time I would go in a nursing home – if I got dirty. I couldn't stick it ... you know I couldn't stand it."

Another woman also experienced the transfer as a loss, but was able to alleviate this because she could afford to employ her own private help:

Mrs Burford is a widow of 80. She was very sorry to lose her home carers:

> "Well they were really lovely, I could trust them, I couldn't have had better people.... They were lovely – they still send Christmas cards and things like that. It was a real loss."

However, she expressed her understanding that "there was so many people waiting for them that the nursing – the home nursing – came first, which I can quite understand."

She was also happy with the help she got from HITH: "They sent me a very good person and she did one hour's ironing and one hour's shopping for me". However, the home assistant left and, while it is a policy of the service to ensure shopping is done, HITH were unable to provide someone to do her ironing. Mrs Burford has quite severe osteoporosis and cannot manage this herself. She therefore employed her HITH assistant in a private capacity for shopping and ironing.

Mrs Burford did not find HITH as flexible as home care:

> "I think always with the home carers, if one couldn't come for some reason, always somebody else came in their place which it doesn't always apply for [HITH]. They'd send somebody, they wouldn't see me without any shopping, but they couldn't always spare anybody for the ironing."

For Mrs Burford, losing her home carers was one of a series of cumulative losses. Her husband had died in the period immediately before the transfer and her sister-in-law, with whom she had a close relationship, died shortly after. She was, though, in her own terms, more fortunate than many other older people in that she was able to afford to pay for help. This she did extensively, including a private cleaner whom she had employed for five years. She described this woman as "like a daughter to me" and to some extent this appeared to provide a continuity of feeling cared about as well as ensuring the upkeep of her home.

It is not insignificant that all three women used familial terms when describing their relationships with their 'formal' helpers. Using the language of 'daughter', as did other older participants, indicates an emotional closeness based on reciprocal caring (Wenger, 1992). There was little doubt that for some of our older participants, home carers 'replaced' the daughters they did not have or who lived some distance away. For some other older people, the intrinsic value of the help was more friendship than familial-based. Mrs Styles, for example, said that having a chat with Betty and "the girls" was "a bit of therapy". Betty herself put it so:

> "You're not to get involved, that's one of the things they say, you must not get involved. That's fine but when you're going into somebody day after day, week after week, you get to know them and you know when they're upset – you know, when things are not going right for them. You know and you try to be helpful, don't you? And try to cheer them up, you know. And they say you mustn't do this sort of thing. I mean at one time you weren't allowed to sit down and have a cup of tea but sometimes that's what people want you to do."

It seemed that for the women the instrumental value of the help received was interwoven with the intrinsic benefits. Those older female participants who had developed closer relationships with their home carers were also often those who were pleased about the standard of the housework performed. That home carers often did little extras – like taking net curtains home and washing them – indicated that they understood the value of the appearance of the home to their clients. This mutual understanding undoubtedly contributed to their relationship.

Starting with independent sector help

We should point out that where older people started with help from independent sector providers, including HITH, their perceptions of the value of those services were often quite different to the initial responses of the people transferred. Mrs Simpson, for example, who accessed HITH directly, said the service met her needs for help with housework and that because the home assistants were carefully vetted she felt she could trust them. Trust was stated by a number of our participants as a crucial factor. For some, it meant turning to 'reputable' organisations but for many, as indicated above, it was also about relationships developed with formal carers. Many older participants told us that they would prefer to be able to manage alone and it seems that it's just 'easier' if they are able to develop a friendship with people who are coming into their lives and homes.

Moving into higher levels of need

Two of our city participants initially transferred to HITH were later moved back to the SSD but at a higher level of provision. In both cases, there was arguably a lack of recognition of the wider needs of the older person.

Mrs Ellis is a widow of 88. She has a large supportive family but all her friends have died. She had been a client of home care/home help for 10 years when she was transferred to HITH. She needed personal assistance but being "extremely modest" would only allow her granddaughter to help her in this because she was a nurse. Mrs Ellis' son died two years ago and she is still grieving for him. This undoubtedly contributed to her low feelings which were clear sometimes during our interviews with her. She had had her home carer – Mary – for six years and had established the sort of relationship whereby Mary had become "more of a friend" who "knew all the family". Mary was about the same age as her late son and Mrs Ellis found losing Mary very difficult:

> "Well I was really upset really. 'Cos I mean – it's when you're older dear, you need someone to come in and help you.... It's when you're feeling bad you want someone round. You feel as though you're on your own and it's an awful feeling when you're old and there's nobody there you can call."

Mrs Ellis found HITH more expensive than home care and this was clearly an issue for her. More than this, her first HITH assistant had, in her terms, "mucked up ... she came for two weeks and then left". She was then given a young male assistant, who she said was "very nice" but "they're not running it like the home help service". Part of this related to the time-keeping of her assistant, part related to the fact that there was no cover over Christmas:

"I mean at Christmas, two weeks off. Well! It's when you're older you want someone to come in and do the work for you."

Mrs Ellis also didn't like to say what she wanted done:

"He says 'What do I want done?' I don't like telling people what to do. I like them to get on with it – Mary used to get straight on. She used to know."

When we visited Mrs Ellis six months later she told us that she now had an independent provider coming in, organised by social services. Her HITH assistant had left and Mrs Ellis had been without help for three weeks. Her medical condition had deteriorated and she had developed psoriasis. Her daughter contacted social services and requested an assessment for her mother. This was duly done and Mrs Ellis was assessed as being in need of 'personal care' – she needed cream applied to her back for her psoriasis. She still only allows her granddaughter intimate access but now receives her service free of charge for half an hour, five mornings a week, plus an additional two hours one morning a week. This is nominally for bathing but is used in reality for housework.

It was the opinion of the present care manager that the transfer from home care had failed to take Mrs Ellis' grieving into account and that it indicated a lack of understanding of depression and mental health problems. It was the care manager's view that Mrs Ellis was depressed because of her son's death and although she admitted it was impossible to link Mrs Ellis' medical condition to the transfer, she did point out:

"I mean I'm back now paying an agency to do exactly the same as they were doing. So what good was that? Why did they do it?"

Mrs Wright is 86 and lives alone. She had home care since 1989 following a period of hospitalisation with a heart problem. Mrs Wright now has osteoarthritis and breast cancer. She was unable to go out alone, was lonely and didn't "have many people come in to see me for a chat". In fact, she had only one person visiting her once a fortnight who helped her with shopping.

She was transferred to HITH because her service was based upon housework and shopping only. Yet she told us that her home carer did occasionally wash her hair, as this was something she had "great difficulty with". She had had her home carer for some time, and although she does not seem to have developed a particular friendship with her, she was upset about the change because: "Well you got used to the people, you know?"

Mrs Wright did not feel that she had any choice in the transfer: "Well I just had to ... you got to accept it, 'cos you're old and you've got to have some help, you see". She was, however, worried about its impact:

> "Well getting people to get the things to do 'cos I can't get out at all and things like you ... when you want a stamp and that ... and all that sort of thing. That's the worry of it."

She also said that her condition had "got worse" since the transfer and she now had more difficulty both in washing her hair and ensuring her own level of personal hygiene. These concerns were matched by worries about her receding energy levels and her ability to perform housework tasks:

> "Well I'm getting ... I've found ... today, I had to do this ironing 'cos she [the home assistant] took me washing over to the launderette yesterday, you see. And I dried it in here and I had to iron it and I found it really ... I was nearly exhausted time I'd finished. That it was too much, you know. It worries me 'cos I don't know whether I shall have to go in a home or not. I don't want to go in a home ... if I can help it."

For Mrs Wright, it was cooking for herself that stood between staying at home and going into residential care:

> "Well that I couldn't get to me dinner ... doing me dinners and things like that. I should ... I should have to do something then."

We asked Mrs Wright if she was aware that she could go back to social services and request more help. She clearly found this difficult to contemplate. On the one hand, she found it difficult to ask for help saying that she felt it would mean she was being "a nuisance to other people". On the other, she was not convinced that she could get a service: "No, I don't think so, 'cos it's altogether different now. They sort of cast me off from there".

When we visited Mrs Wright again six months later, we found that she was now receiving help from a private agency, organised by social services. She had asked her home assistant for help with a strip wash. This is outside HITH's remit and therefore Mrs Wright was referred back to social services for an assessment. At that stage an hour's assistance each evening with washing/bathing and meal preparation was organised.

Shortly afterwards, however, Mrs Wright contacted social services saying that she could manage alone and wanted the service withdrawn. The care manager told us that she had had to visit Mrs Wright several times before she would accept that she needed help. She also told us Mrs Wright had been unhappy with the arrangement because she found that it disrupted her preferred evening schedule. The care manager then asked the agency manager to do a hands-on assessment for a couple of days.

At that stage it was realised that Mrs Wright liked to prepare her own meals, although the care manager still seemed unaware that this was what Mrs Wright perceived as standing between her and 'a home': that this was her boundary insofar as maintaining her independence was concerned. Both professionals had some concern about her safety in preparing food and therefore decided that support should be there while she did so. Nevertheless, for Mrs Wright, the outcome was good. She appreciates the company:

> "Well it helps 'cos you got somebody to talk to. They're very good – they do quite a lot. I mean I can get me dinner – they send her really to get me dinner and that, but I can do that meself. I can manage that meself. It's getting on about ... I can't move me furniture or anything.... Well anything I wants done."

Rural areas: home help – bulk versus spot purchasing

In the rural area, senior SSD professionals told us that they had managed to retain the home help service by taking up the slack in home carer hours. They would, they said, prefer to target in-house services upon older people "with the most intensive personal care needs". The stated reasons for this were two-fold. Firstly, the SSD has a legal mandate and therefore a stronger foundation to provide the services themselves; secondly, independent sector providers sometimes lack the requisite experience to deal with "vulnerable people and complex family situations". The corollary would be to transfer those people with primarily domestic assistance needs to independent providers. However, they pointed to the problems in developing independent sector provision in rural areas where time and travelling costs are higher. Spot purchasing, they said, undermined business stability for would-be providers and could impact upon quality in part because of poorer employment conditions.

These factors mean that not only is 'vulnerability' a factor in assessment but so too is geographical area. This particular SSD is committed to stimulating more varied provision by encouraging independent sector involvement through bulk purchasing. Again, however, the professionals told us that this can be inefficient and difficult to manage, and that it was a field in which they needed to develop more expertise. They were clear, though, that any transfer of older people to the independent sector had to be carefully handled, recognising that there could be long-term detrimental effects if the process discouraged the active involvement of older people:

> "If people don't take part actively in that process, they feel things are done to them. It's a known factor in tailing off levels of help, and it's not in our interests to do that because people can deteriorate and have their emotional stability taken away." (service manager)

4

The importance of safety and social participation

Feeling safe

Getting unknown people to help in their homes can be threatening to older people. A couple of older participants told us that they would not employ cleaners from cards in shop windows because "You can't vet them, can you? You don't know who you're going to get into your house". It seemed that, for the women in particular, there was considerable concern about having unknown men in their homes. Sometimes the concern was about being over-charged for work, of being "taken advantage of because you're old"; sometimes it seemed more the threat of attack and/or robbery. With such a sensitive topic we refrained from probing too deeply as we did not wish to create or heighten fear. It was very clear, though, that our older participants preferred to use reputable organisations for the repair and maintenance of their homes. As Mrs Chase put it:

> "Elderly people are afraid to pick up the paper and see 'odd job man' and get him in; you don't know who you're getting in, do you? There's an awful lot of fear with elderly people. There is with me."

Mrs Miles turned to Care and Repair when she had a problem with her front door. She was advised that she needed rather more work done to her house and, with the help of Care and Repair, secured a grant to refit her kitchen and to install an upstairs bathroom. She was delighted with the outcome and felt confident to go out while the work was going on to avoid the mess.

Mrs Chase also got help from Care and Repair to secure a minor works grant and to organise the work involved in replacing her windows, without which she said she would have been unable to remain in her home:

"Having these windows done was very important to me, yes, to stay here because they were eventually going to fall out ... and I would have had to sell up."

Like others who received help from this organisation, Mrs Chase felt confident because "It's nice to know if you're getting someone in they're coming from a reputable organisation".

Mrs Griffiths similarly felt safe with the Care and Repair Handyperson scheme:

"Care and Repair are the only people I have here. I have Colin, he does all the odd-jobs ... he's honest ... he knows all the jobs, he does them to perfection. He's the only one I have in here.... He knows how to do everything – housewise."

Getting window cleaners posed particular problems for some older people who found it impossible to get this help. For others living in high rise flats the only way of getting the windows cleaned was to have the male window cleaner come into the flat. One residents group found an innovative solution in consultation with the window cleaner, however. His wife now accompanies him and the added bonus for the older residents is that she will change their curtains.

Security: locks, bolts and alarms

The loss of a partner in later life can leave older people feeling vulnerable. For one woman this was exacerbated by her deafness. She developed her own coping strategy but came to realise that this in fact increased her vulnerability.

Mrs Allen was a widow in her 80s, living alone. She described herself as "completely helpless" without her hearing aid. She had had a number of specialist alarms and security locks fitted following her husband's death three years before and a period in hospital. She also had a pendant alarm and her neighbours had the keys to get into the bungalow in case of emergency.

In the time between her husband's death and getting this help, Mrs Allen had a friend fit bolts to the inside of her bedroom door because she was "scared, having never been alone in a house before in my life. I was really frightened." Since getting her pendant alarm she could no longer use these bolts because of access. Mrs Allen feels safer with the alarms and locks but:

> "It's not like when my husband was alive. I didn't have to worry about hearing any noises ... I could go to sleep and I knew if anything happened he would deal with it. Now I can't hear thunder and lightning."

Mrs Allen missed her husband terribly. They were married for 55 years – "a lifetime really" – and his death had been a shock.

> "It's a terrible thing, you know, he's gone. I can sit here and talk to you or anybody who comes in, have a good old natter. But you know you're watching the football in the evening, you've got no one to comment to. I never thought I'd be left alone, with all my aches and pains. I thought I'd be gone long before Bob. It's such a shock, really."

Mrs Allen's situation also suggests the 'dripping tap' syndrome where the loss of her partner led to feeling unsafe. Although the alarms and security devices could not engender the same sense of security as when her husband was alive, they were still valuable to her.

In the conurbation case study area, older people can get home safety devices through a 'safe city' project. Mrs Caldwell, an 81-year-old widow, was offered this service following a fall which led to a stay in hospital. Mrs Caldwell said that at that time "they" rather than she thought the fitting of safety locks necessary. At first she declined, but later thought that she "really ought to have it done", particularly as it had been suggested to her that she might otherwise be penalised over her house contents insurance. Although she had not been worried about the locks at the time, her response to a question about whether they made her feel safer was as follows:

> "Yes I do, yes I think that's as I've got older because I've had them two or three years now and I feel safer each year if that makes sense."

A second case study also highlights the value of locks and bolts to older people:

> Mrs Fisher, a widow of 82, came into the safe city scheme following an attempted break-in at her bungalow. Before that she had never felt nervous, but the attempted burglary had threatened to undermine this. However, the fitting of catches on her windows and doors had allowed her to re-establish her own sense of safety:
>
> > "I'm quite happy about it all now and the two doors – the last things that I had done, quite recently – that has been marvellous. They are very good doors, wonderful bolts on them. I was reasonably happy about it, and those catches on the windows helped so much and especially on the door, the side door, so that people can't get into the garden."
>
> Mrs Fisher said that she had now been able to resume a normal life:
>
> > "I've even surprised myself. Not that I've ever been a 'sit at home' but even so, one is justified in being a little worried, especially with what you hear these days – what younger people do to old people. I'm more shocked than frightened, I can tell you."

Fear of crime

A number of our older participants talked about their fear of crime outside as well as inside the home. Mrs Griffiths, a widow in her mid-70s, talked about her loneliness, which she described as "a killer". A number of break-ins in her area had led her to have locks fitted to the inner doors of her house as well as to the external ones and windows by a local policeman friend. This strategy, however, had in effect reduced her feelings of well-being: "It's driving me bloody mad, locked in, barred in, bolted in here".

At the same time, she was afraid to go out. She had been widowed for many years and more recent losses of friends had undoubtedly increased her feelings of isolation.

For Mrs Griffiths, it was not so much services she needed. Rather, "I need something to do. I need someone to say 'get your glad rags on.'" She said that there were a lot of older people like her – "fit, agile and lonely" – for whom day centres and lunch clubs were not the answer to their need "for a purpose to live." She would have liked to be able to go to social events in the evening but her fear of being attacked and the lack of 'reputable transport' made this impossible. Instead she felt barricaded in her house without safe alternatives and she was, in her own terms, severely depressed.

Mrs Fisher, who had managed the tension between feeling secure within her house and having the freedom to go out, nevertheless felt constrained by social attitudes. These were reminiscent of those which focus upon the behaviour of women who are victims of crime and thereby restrict women's freedom of movement, but with the added the dimension of age:

> "I must be back at sixish, as most elderly people are, some of whom hardly go out let alone get back. I never would stay out really late, 'cos I don't want people to say of me: 'Silly old women, out late'. I don't know – it's that little added 'old', isn't it?"

A preventative strategy against fear of crime and social isolation

In the city area, there is increasing recognition that older people's fear of crime – widely recognised as out of sync with actual risk – may be mitigated by greater social integration. It is felt that the social isolation of many older people intensifies their fear of crime and levels of depression. Not only is their quality of life reduced, but their ability to care for themselves is undermined. Realisation on the part of the city council that there is a correlation between social isolation and fear of crime led to the allocation of crime prevention money to the development team at the SSD to develop local level initiatives to reduce both. At the time of writing, a number of initiatives were being planned. These included encouraging intergenerational contact, reintroducing good neighbour schemes, and collating information about local services and facilities with the active involvement of community centres.

According to an SSD development worker who has a central role in coordinating this initiative at local level:

"It is one of a number of ways of focusing upon the problem. I mean obviously there are practical things like saying 'This is the reality of what the risks are and these are ways you can make yourself safer' by fitting door locks, by getting the home security service. There is a role to play I think for the police in actually talking to groups of older people about 'Well actually you are at very low risk'. It's about the reality of the situation and trying to defuse the anxiety but also it's about quality of life issues. And I think if you talk to your neighbours, if you have enough services to maximise your independence and so on, you're much less likely to view crime as problematic than if you're isolated and you're behind your locked doors."

This would appear to be a valuable preventative strategy in the making. Yet perhaps it again requires recognition of a gender dimension in that social isolation is more commonly an issue for women than men. More than this, however, as the development worker recognised, availability of the requisite level of services to maximise independence is a crucial variable. The importance of domiciliary services demands emphasis here.

Social outlets

Luncheon clubs, coffee mornings, day centres and so on can provide both the opportunity for company and for the dissemination of information among older people about what help is available. There was a range of such facilities, though more in the urban than the rural areas, which were run by SSDs, the voluntary sector, churches and community centres/groups. Apart from SSD day centres, the voluntary staff comprised mostly older people and at least two we visited were organised by older people: one aged 65, the other 93.

When we asked at one luncheon club what was most valued, the answer was the 'company of friends' and the chance to reminisce. Others stressed the importance of "getting out of the house". One of our participants, Mrs Miles, also welcomed the meal: she was finding it increasingly difficult to cook for herself, being afraid of splashing herself with fat. She also told us, however, that she attends all possible social facilities "else I sits here hours and hours on me own. I do get fed up with meself at times".

These facilities did not meet the needs of all our participants, however. For some, they were simply "not my cup of tea". For others they were "too cliquey" or lacking in intellectual stimulation. Transport was mentioned by some as problematic, particularly in the rural area for older people who would have liked to attend daytime social facilities. Mrs Cox was able to attend the occasional coffee morning run by a local club when her daughter could take her there by car, but Mrs Norris was unable to attend because "I don't like to ask for a lift". She wished someone would be "kind enough to offer".

5
Themes and issues

Not having to ask

Among the benefits of low level preventative services was that they provided an alternative to having to ask the family. The majority of our older participants said that they found asking for help from *anyone* difficult. Mrs Moss, for example, did not like to ask her neighbours for help unless she really had to. She saw asking as akin to "giving in" which itself threatened her independence. Where help was accepted from neighbours, this tended to be for shopping and pension collection and was usually part of a reciprocal relationship, involving exchange of food, gifts, looking out for one another or simply providing mutual comfort. Help with housework did not generally come into this exchange.

Continuity in terms of who is coming in to the home might also be stressed here. Some of our older participants did not want to have to ask the 'carer' to do this or that. They much preferred the situation where the carer knew what to do. Mrs Moss pointed out: "I prefer a regular girl. They know the routine. They know exactly ... we get a routine between us".

Developing "a routine between us" indicates active involvement rather than passive receipt which undoubtedly mitigated the feeling of 'giving in' and therefore the loss of independence. This was further protected when home carers did little extras without the older person having to ask: "I didn't ask them, they offered".

That's not to say that all our older participants found it easy to accept help. Mrs Moon put it so:

> "I've always liked doing things for myself. I mean, if somebody said 'I'll help you' I said 'no, it's alright'. Sometimes you need a little bit of help ... but I wouldn't like to be clobbered down, getting everybody to do everything for me. I would struggle on rather than ask."

Mrs Smith believed that older people better understand the importance of being offered help rather than having to ask for it:

> "The young ones – they sympathise with you but they wouldn't say, well.... Other people are kind, don't get me wrong. But the *older* people, they got the sense enough to say, well ... immediately help you. 'Cos I expect we all think the same. We may be in the same boat – need a bit of help. Which, when you're down, you do need a bit of help, don't you?"

She distinguished between people who said "just pick up the phone and 'let us know' " and those who offered, on the grounds "that's the help they want to give you".

Some forms of help were easier to accept. The laundry service run by the large voluntary organisation in the city was particularly appreciated and incurred no loss of independence. Mrs Reid, for example, said it was "very good ... because I've only got a washboy, that's all I've got so it comes in very useful for me, see, to send it to the laundry." When asked if she got any other form of help, she replied "No, no, I don't want to feel I'm too old to do anything, not at the moment. I'm 81 but I keep going ... no, otherwise I'm alright."

Mrs Foster, who has severe arthritis in her hands, described the same service as "the best thing that ever happened for older people". Both she and Mrs Reid lived in a high rise where lack of a garden made drying washing extremely difficult. For Mrs Foster, the service also meant that there was an alternative to relying upon her daughters although they were very supportive and helped her out a great deal. Having endured a long marriage to a violent husband who had subjected the family to poverty, however, she would have liked to be the one helping:

> "I do worry about things, I can't help it. I'm trying to make up to my daughters for what I was never able to give them when they were little. I always give them love and that, they know that but ... erm 'Oh mum, you don't have to do that, it's us that'll do for you'".

Alternatives to asking the family

Getting 'a bit of help in' was seen as preferable for many to asking families for help. For those in the city aware of the voluntary organisation's Help in the Home (HITH) scheme, this was the source they did or would turn to for help with housework. Families did provide help to some of our older participants but, for others, the fact that their sons and daughters lived some way away made this rather piecemeal. Also, of course, there were participants who had no immediate family, which was discussed as a matter of regret.

Asking the family for help seemed to amount sometimes to an admission of not coping in the face of family concerns that they indeed could not cope. Mrs Black told us that her daughter had said that "You can't go on like this mother. You shouldn't be climbing ladders, you shouldn't be doing that. Why don't you ask me?" Mrs Black said she wouldn't ask them for help because "They've got to have their life. I'm independent. I'd rather be like that than go running to anybody". Mrs Moon similarly said that her daughter sometimes says "Mother, you can't do that" but that she didn't like "people doing things" for her. When she had a fall in her garden she asked her neighbours not to let her children know because she thought "Oh, they're gonna start 'You can't do this and that' again."

A number of older people talked about their families being busy and having their own lives to lead and it was within this context that the term 'burden' was used most often. This is applied 'frequently and freely' to older people and carries with it a dichotomy of strength and weakness in, respectively, care-giving and care-receiving relationships (Warnes, 1993). On the one hand, the 'burden of caring' is borne by the care-giver; on the other, the care-recipient becomes a burden. Our older participants did not want to be 'burdens' to their families. They felt it was not only their own independence which was undermined by this, so too was that of their families.

As we shall discuss below, definitions of independence shifted. Yet at the core was the retention of choice and control. It is within this sense that we understand how our older participants viewed having to ask the family as a threat not only to their own but also to their families' independence. On numerous occasions our older participants pointed out that it was unfair to always ask their families. This was tempered by their own wish to manage and to be seen to manage for themselves. As one woman stated: "I don't want to be a burden to anybody, I would rather struggle on, struggle on myself and get a little bit of help in".

Although family support was appreciated, there were mixed feelings at times. Mrs Malone said of daughters: "You can't beat them, can you?" At the same time though, much of the value she accorded her services was based upon the fact that if somebody else did it, her daughter wouldn't have to. She also said that her daughter "loses her patience with me sometimes". When asked about how that happens, she tearfully replied: "Well you know, sometimes you sit and sigh and think 'Oh I'm fed up with this' and they don't like you saying it, you know".

Mrs Chase described a community gardening service as

> "a Godsend to me 'cos if I want anything now in the garden, I don't have to bother them, do I? I like my family to have their own independence. I don't want to be an obligation to them. I don't want to be calling on them for Dick, Tom and Harry. If I can possibly get by meself, I will, and that's a Godsend to me because once in six months I can find £6 to get my garden straightened up, can't I?.... It's a great help to elderly people if they've got a garden, but nobody knows about it. You see, you don't know these things. This is what I don't understand."

Mrs Chase said that her daughter tended to be a bit 'bossy' and to interfere. She also said she had asked her daughter to wipe round her window frames but that she had "not got round to it". Nor had she, despite a number of requests, helped to pull the bed out so Mrs Chase could clean behind it. Undoubtedly her daughter would bring a different perspective to the story. However, the point is that the rhetoric of community care policy – that families want to help – does not recognise how difficult it can be to ask for help from the older person's point of view and how what they perceive as a rejection may serve to reinforce feelings of dependency. Although family help was appreciated, it was most appreciated when it was offered and many of our older people said quite clearly that they didn't like to ask. For instance, Mrs Marks said:

"It's much nicer if people offer than to be always asking, but people don't seem to know that, that's the trouble. It's the independence of me and people like me against people that aren't over-willing, and you've got this constant rub. You see, if they were more easy-going you could ask them and then you wouldn't have this independence thing, but they put you into this independence thing."

Help or care

It is clear that, for many of our participants, the assistance they get is supportive of their wish to do as much as possible for themselves. Along with staying in their own homes, which enables choice and control, taking care of themselves has been most commonly mentioned as central to their feelings of independence. Our older participants were determined to protect their independence and were prepared, though sometimes reluctantly, to get in 'a little bit of help' to support that:

"You can't be *too* independent, can you, when you need help? No. But it does help me to be independent – it doesn't stop you from being independent."

"Now, I prefer to be in my own home and, you know, look after myself as much as I possibly can *with* that bit of help".

Whether our older participants talked about help with housework, personal assistance, house and garden maintenance or security, they called it *help,* not *care.* Although some of those older people in receipt of home care referred to a carer, these people too still talked about the service as help. Mrs Styles said of the personal and domestic assistance she received:

"I know I've got to rely on them because I can't do it myself, I've got to rely on them and I don't feel that I'm losing my independence with them."

Mrs Moss similarly said that the assistance helps her cope. We asked her whether getting things done for her took away her independence. She replied:

"No, not one little bit, no ... well it helps me to be able to *cope*. It helps me to cope, really, because you know, when you can't bend or lift, anything like that and you know that somebody's going to come and do it for you."

When asked what made it possible to retain her independence, she replied:

"All the time I can get help. All the time I *know* I can get that help – or that I can get more if I want it. If they stop the home help, I just couldn't stay here. There's no way I could stay here. For one thing, I couldn't get out. And I couldn't manage the house. That is just the home help – home care.... And I know the girls will be in – I know somebody will be in. It's that independence that I will be able to say 'Well I know the girls are coming in tomorrow – I'll be OK'."

Help has quite a different meaning to care (Morris, 1993). For our older participants, care implied being looked after and consequently the *loss* of independence. Mrs Callaghan said:

"You see I've always had to think for myself and depend on myself. So I suppose it's made me more independent, when you have to make your own decisions and stand or fall by them. But ... perhaps other people just want to be looked after, but I haven't got to that stage yet."

When we asked Mrs Callaghan whether or not the help she got with housework was care or support, she replied:

"I suppose it's support to help me care for myself. 'Cos I couldn't look after this flat, well I could but it would get a bit tatty you know. I would have to get help from somewhere else."

That older people talk about help rather than care is somewhat different to professional discourses on the subject. Here we found a recurrent tendency to define people who were perceived as having high level needs as 'dependent' per se. 'Independence' was thereby reduced to the ability to perform what are perceived as the essential activities of daily living. Professionals countered our challenge to this by stating that it didn't matter what terms they used as long as the service was delivered.

However, while SSDs have a statutory responsibility to meet the needs of people who meet eligibility criteria, those same people may also be in receipt of low level preventative services like housework which are bolted on to their personal assistance. Moreover, cost ceilings operate in such a way as to limit the amount of low level service input: the greater the intensity of personal assistance, the lesser can be the intensity of low level assistance. This can leave those older people with significant levels of impairment with rather less domestic help than they need and which they feel is central to the maintenance of their independence.

In the city, some of our participants who were in receipt of home care talked about how they really needed more help with housework. However, they were excluded from the HITH scheme because this would mean "the service would have been very quickly bunged up with people needing a lot of care and there were other ways of providing their care." It would seem, then, that being in receipt of statutory services, and thus carrying with them the label of dependency, excludes older people from some preventative services; instead they are perceived as needing care at the expense of help with the tasks that are important to them. The definition of dependency is more than a mere operational term; its consequences are very real. As they seek to meet their statutory obligations, professionals involved in policy formulation may be in danger of losing sight of what is really important to older people regardless of their level of functional impairment.

Transgressing professional boundaries

The intrinsic value older people derive from low level services comprises for many the emotional benefits of feeling cared about and knowing someone is there 'just in case'. Such benefits have been widely identified as enhancing health and well-being (Sidell, 1997), and they are those that older people give up only reluctantly (Gray, 1988). Professionals away from the front line of provision are sometimes critical of home carers and others who 'transgress' professional boundaries by forming personal relationships and acting outside their remit.

There is, of course, a range of issues involved. In one area, there had been some considerable difficulties over gifts and people leaving property in wills. Concern was also expressed that it is not possible to guarantee that a particular carer will always be there for any one older person: geographical patches are changed, carers come and go. Indeed a HITH coordinator told us that they now had the same 'problem' when their clients were transferred to high level statutory support.

Professional boundaries are also there to protect formal carers. We have witnessed the distress of individual home carers when clients have died, and some welcome a periodic change in their individual client groups to shield their level of involvement and feelings. As one service manager said the danger is that "staff sometimes cannot disentangle themselves from the world of that person's life". There is no simple either/or here because providing assistance in people's homes is ipso facto involvement in their lives and relationships do develop between formal care-givers and care-recipients.

Enhancing or undermining independence?

Mrs Ashton is 84; her husband was 81. They got daily home care. It was difficult at first to decipher whom the service was for, as Mr Ashton was ill in bed and Mrs Ashton had her leg in plaster. In fact the service was targeted at Mr Ashton who had leukaemia although Mrs Ashton believed it was for her. She did, however, have a respite sitting service. The sitter undertook a range of tasks which Mrs Ashton couldn't do herself including taking curtains down, cleaning high shelves, taking parcels to the post and helping her bath. The home carers prepared lunch every day for the couple and did housework, shopping and pension collection. Mrs Ashton had had pneumonia three years earlier and at that point Mr Ashton had become the main care-giver, taking over most of the household tasks including those now done by home care and the sitter.

Mrs Ashton enjoyed all the company she got from these services, most particularly the conversation. She found it difficult to sustain a conversation with her husband who was quite deaf and she had very little contact with other people. It was also important to her that there was someone there to "keep an eye" on them. The affective value was very important to Mrs Ashton. One of 'the girls', she said, "kisses me on the side of my face – I can't get over it!" She liked this, saying it was "nice."

Mr Ashton died in hospital three months after our first meeting and we visited Mrs Ashton again three months later. Both sets of services had been withdrawn and Mrs Ashton was now getting help from HITH with her housework. She told us that she now had to "struggle" to have a bath and feel safe: "I have to put a towel down inside. When I get out I have to wait till the bath runs out, put a towel down to stand on it to pull myself up at the sides". She said that she would like somebody to be there to make sure she could get out of the bath safely and thought she might arrange her bath times to coincide with the home assistant's visits so that "she can see that I can get out".

One might think that Mrs Ashton would be likely to be referred back to social services. However, her former care manager had a less than positive view of the relationship between Mrs Ashton and the sitter:

> "That carer had got very, very close to her – it was almost a friendship – and was doing things that she hadn't been asked to do. The sitting service was supposed to be giving respite but she was taking a whole parcel of goodness knows what else which wasn't really a part of her remit. I think she was trying to be as kind as she possibly could but not understanding that she was making this poor lady dependent."

The care manager's perception following the reassessment was that Mrs Ashton's husband had "pampered her" and that Mrs Ashton "had got into this letting other people do things for her". Her fear had been that Mrs Ashton "had really made herself dependent and as far as I'm concerned we weren't doing her favours if we continued with the care". She said that Mrs Ashton "had the ability to be far more self-caring than she herself realised". She had no second thoughts about the advisability of withdrawing the service, but did this "gradually to ease it down to make her more self-reliant." The care manager was aware that the sitter was helping Mrs Ashton bathe but felt that "she should be able to do it herself". She also told us that she had made Mrs Ashton aware that "if she had any worries that she wasn't 'coping' she could get back in touch with us."

However, some problems arise from these perceptions and actions. For Mrs Ashton, part of the value of the services she received was that they helped her "to survive until I can do it myself" and that she "would prefer to cope on my own". She said that she dreaded of the thought of going into a home and was therefore prepared to get as much help as possible to enable her to stay in her own home. Mrs Ashton did not feel she could manage without help but did not see that help as undermining her independence. Her ideas about independence were then completely different to those of the care manager. At the same time, Mrs Ashton was having to make major role transitions in adjustment to living alone and dealing with the finances and the maintenance of the home. She was in fact very grateful for the information leaflets we gave her on Handyperson services having recently paid a great deal of money to a plumber in her terms "for nothing".

Shifting boundaries of independence

Our older participants clearly did not equate the need for assistance with dependency. Not only did they describe assistance as help to self-care, they shifted their boundaries of what comprised independence in line with their changing capacities and other circumstances. Capacities, of course, can increase as well as decrease.

Mrs Smith had already reduced her home care. She received, among other things, assistance with washing but found that she could do that for herself again. She was concerned that if she came to rely too heavily on the services she would lose the capacity to do things for herself:

> "I've always been independent, very independent. And I feel if I come to rely ... rely on somebody, I'm going to become an invalid and I shall be forever wanting somebody helping me."

She also phased out the evening help with preparation for bed because the carer came at 7pm which was too early for her:

> "I was really wild. 7 o'clock! I mean, I'd barely got me tea and washed up. I said 'I'm not bed-ridden thankfully. Putting my bottle up at this time of night is ridiculous. I'm afraid I shall be phasing you people out.'"

Mrs Smith eventually decided to phase out her weekday assistance – she said that her days revolved around home care so much that she was worried she would become "housebound" and "I would become dependent – well, I couldn't afford that – I'm too young at 82." She wanted, however, to retain her laundry service and weekend meal delivery but was told that she could not have these unless she had 'personal care'. Mrs Smith said she was "hurt" by social services' response:

> "... they care? They say they care! And that got at me. I thought to meself well, where's the caring in that? They knew what pain I was in and yet under my *own steam* to get out – away from them – I would have been quite happy for them to still go me bit. ... Because I didn't have the carers, I couldn't have the other perks. Well, I don't call that caring at all. So, if at some future date – which I hope there won't be – I hope I pass on, to be honest with you – at some future date I've got to have care, I will not go back to *them*. No! It hurt me and I expect it's hurt other people. Where's the caring in that?"

Mrs Smith referred herself to HITH. She had previously had advice from the parent organisation and had found them "very helpful ... *that's* the caring". She was thereby able to re-access the laundry service and we gave her information about meal delivery services. One point that might be made here is that if Mrs Smith had been caring for someone else, she would have probably got her services from the SSD. It was because she wanted to self-care that she could not. She had, according to the professionals, got better and therefore neither needed nor qualified for statutory support. This may reflect the rules but it points to a lack of flexibility in low level service provision.

The following case studies provide two further examples of the fluidity of the concept of independence and how people redefine their perceptions of themselves as independent beings.

Mrs Jones first 'shifted her boundaries' when she moved into sheltered accommodation. She felt she could no longer manage her house and was nervous living alone after her husband died: "I thought this isn't on and I need to go somewhere where it'd be better". She didn't consult her family about the move because "I'm a little bit independent".

When we asked her what she meant by independence, she replied:

> "Well I like to be able to cope on my own as long as I can and as well as I can. That is my independence. I mean people are helpful but at the same time I still want to know I can do what they want to do for me."

The help she now needed with hoovering and laundry didn't undermine that "... because I need it. That I can give up 'cos I know I can't do it."

Mrs Jones' capacities to perform certain tasks have decreased with deterioration in her medical condition. What would threaten her independence is to have someone do the things she can still do for herself. She was able to do her own shopping with the assistance of local taxi-drivers. Retaining this was vital to her:

> "...don't take that away from me. All the time I can go up the shops and do what I want shop-wise ... all the time I'm able to do that, I'm independent. My independence is when I say 'I can do that myself, I don't need you to do it'."

For Mrs Allen, as with some other women, independence was about cooking her own meals:

> "I'm reluctant to go in a home yet because I'm still able to do some things, I can please meself what I do. I think the time to go into a home is when you can't cook for yourself."

She told us that a friend who had recently died had let herself go down such that "she couldn't cook for herself" although she had kept "her place very nice". When we first met Mrs Allen she had told us that she might need some help in the future but she wasn't sure what she could get and therefore was concerned she might have to "give up" her bungalow. We gave her numerous information leaflets. Some months later, she had a fall and directly accessed HITH but only for help with the tasks she couldn't manage alone:

> "I was just getting to the stage when I thought, well I can't ... I thought I'd better give it up, but now I know I've got someone to rely on, I'm, you know, more able to think 'Well, yeah. I'll go on a bit longer!'"

For both women, as with so many others, you don't get other people to do for you what you can do yourself. "Use it or lose it" was stressed by a number of participants, as was the importance of willpower. But they did want help to be there and available to them with the things they could *not* manage.

This brings to the fore the old problem about accessing information about what help is available. The research project has acted as a source of information dissemination and older people have indicated how important that is. Even if they feel they don't need any particular form of help at the moment, they want to know it is there 'just in case' – so they don't have to worry *now* about the time they may not be able to manage something in the future.

6

Conclusions and implications

Prevention may be "seen as the very essence of social and community care" (Wistow, 1997, p 2). However, there is a distinct lack of national strategic planning and policy directives concerning low level preventative services.

The impact of targeting is that statutory services are aimed primarily at providing 'care' for people with high level or complex needs. Simply stated, when push comes to shove, statutory agencies will spend their money on personal rather than on domestic assistance. The rationale is that lack of housework is not life-threatening, nor does it stand at the interface of home and institution. However, this report challenges the distinction implied in that rationale between personal assistance and domestic help.

Firstly the differentiation between person (the focus of personal assistance) and environment (the focus of domestic assistance) does not withstand close scrutiny. The home is not simply a physical environment; it can encapsulate the public and private identity of the older person. Their ability to manage the physical environment and be seen to do so impacts upon their well-being and sense of self as a competent adult member of the community. These are crucial factors both in the maintenance of health, function and the ability to adapt to the cumulative losses that ageing can involve and, relatedly, in the social inclusion of older people. There are gender issues here, as discussed in the report, and it may be that further research is needed to investigate the specific needs of men. For the women, however, identity was closely linked to their ability to maintain socially acceptable standards and to retain those domestic tasks that were still within their capacity.

Secondly, there is an implicit, sometimes explicit, assumption that people who need personal assistance are in a different category to people who don't. There is a tendency among professionals to define dependency in terms of the need for personal assistance despite the fact that this is totally out of sync with the perceptions of our older participants. Professionals have claimed that the terms they use matter little as long as the services are delivered. Yet, as this report has demonstrated, the consequences can be very real. On the one hand, older people in receipt of formal personal assistance may receive reduced levels of domestic help as the money and time allocated to their 'category of need' – the cost ceiling – is eaten up by the time and costs of personal assistance. This means they may have to turn to other sources for help with the things that really matter to them. On the other hand, help may be withdrawn from older people with lower levels of need on the grounds that it allegedly encourages dependency.

The importance of domestic help was stressed by all of our older participants, regardless of their 'level of need'. They clearly and consistently stated that the *work* of housework was at least as important as the *care* of personal care. Indeed, the withdrawal of domestic help was perceived by many as indicating social services' lack of understanding and caring about what was important to older people.

During the course of the research we formed the perception, shared by some provider managers, that the low priority given to domestic help reflected the low status which SSDs accorded to housework, which was commonly seen as 'unskilled'. However, this is again out of sync with the perceptions of our older participants, particularly the older women. They had a high regard for the competency and skills involved in housework, and saw access to such help as vital to their ability to retain their independence.

The pressures of targeting and cost-efficiency have led some SSDs to redraw their boundaries of 'core responsibilities' leading to the removal of a solely domestic help service. It may be possible to plug the gap left by this by supporting cost-affordable alternative provision. This research sought to explore to what extent it mattered to older people *who* the provider was, and the report illustrates how one local authority sought to make use of the independent sector. In considering the outcomes for the older people involved, it was clear that it mattered to them that the organisation providing the service was reputable and trustworthy. What was equally clear, however, was the central significance of the relationship developed with the *individual* who was coming in to their home.

Older people often value the intrinsic benefits of feeling cared about as much as they do the help with the task. Indeed the value they give the latter may be inseparable from the relationship with the person performing the task (Henwood et al, 1998). Older people value consistency in terms of who is coming into their homes especially as, for some, this person may be their sole or most significant social contact. Social isolation tends to increase with age as friends and partners die and this can be detrimental to life satisfaction and, relatedly, to mental health (Bowling et al, 1997). The relationship with the front-line provider then takes on added significance. Such issues would be usefully addressed at the level of both policy formulation and practical implementation.

Our older participants perceived independence not in terms of function and deficit, but in terms of staying in their own homes and exercising choice and control. This was the core of independence. At the same time, their definitions of independence were fluid, shifting in line with changing capacities and other circumstances. What could no longer be managed alone could be given up without threatening the core identity of independence.

This would suggest the need for a more flexible and dynamic service response. One way of achieving this would be to allow older people in receipt of statutory support a greater say in how their allocated time/resources are used – in other words, the extension of the principles of independent living to older people. This may be achieved by extending the provision of Direct Payments to older people, who are currently excluded from this under the 1996 Community Care (Direct Payments) Act except in cases of prior receipt. It may also, however, be appropriate to extend the underpinning philosophy of Direct Payments to older people whatever the provisions of the Act, to enable them to exercise choice and control over service provision.

There are, however, more older people outside of SSD services than within, and they may also have a range of needs for support. Low level preventative services may be seen as a way of preventing or delaying their need for statutory support. Many of our older participants organised and financed their own preventative services – which itself indicates their importance – often through known and trusted sources, primarily ex-home-helps/home carers. Others were able to access help from the independent sector.

In the rural area, there were particular difficulties in stimulating independent sector provision (the reliance upon spot purchasing; the high costs of travelling). Consequently, the SSD continued to provide a limited home help service themselves although they were determined to switch to more bulk purchasing to encourage would-be independent providers in the future. Again, however, this would not meet the needs of older people outside of statutory support nor those whose requirements fall outside of core responsibilities. It could be argued that the development of preventative services to provide for older people outside of as well as within statutory support is a challenge for SSDs in general, but for those covering rural areas a range of yet more innovative measures may be necessary (Caldock and Wenger, 1992).

Getting help with home renovation and maintenance was said by some older people to be vital to enabling them to stay in their own homes. They placed great value upon the part played by Care and Repair in organising both the grants and the necessary work. They, along with users of the Care and Repair Handyperson scheme, stressed how important it was to feel safe and confident in terms of both the people coming into their homes and the standard of the work undertaken. Cost-affordability was also highlighted. Similar points were made about help with gardening and again the accessibility of affordable services from reputable organisations was seen as important.

Getting such help meant that they didn't always have to rely upon the family. Older people sometimes have to walk a fine line where family support is concerned. They may appreciate that support but at the same time find it inhibiting of their independence. Not being perceived as a 'burden' and being seen to cope were both stressed as important. Having access to alternative and safe forms of help facilitates this.

Simply knowing the services are there, if and when they're needed, is reassuring to older people and enables them to plan and therefore retain choice and control as their circumstances change.

While older people shift their boundaries of independence, they may perceive some boundaries as unbridgeable or unsustainable in the face of other demands upon their energies and may therefore worry about having to 'give up'. Knowing that help is available before a crisis point is reached and having ready access to that help can make all the difference. 'Knowing' depends upon having information, however, and this can be a problem for older people outside of the network of, for example, luncheon clubs and community centres. The dissemination of information to more isolated older people requires urgent attention.

The policy rhetoric of community care is that care is provided for and to older people in the shape of a mix of formal and informal provision. A number of problematic issues arise from this, not least of which is the presumption that older people are passive recipients of care rather than active agents in their own lives. Our older participants consistently referred to the assistance (whether personal or domestic) they got as *help* rather than care. Help has a different meaning to care, the latter equated to 'being looked after', 'giving in' and consequently the loss of independence. Help, however, was perceived in terms of supporting them to look after themselves and maintain their independence. Again this is an argument for the provision of a range of low level preventative services which are cost-affordable and directly accessible, and which support older people's wish to care for themselves.

The stimulation of a mixed market of low level preventative services is the task facing local authorities. Consideration might be given to ring-fencing of monies for the development of low level services and to protect existing provision against cost-cutting exercises. 'Low level' prevention should not be read as low in value and hence low in priority. These are the services identified by older people as standing between them and residential care. While we have described these services as 'low level' throughout this report, for older people they could equally well be described as 'high value'.

The lack of a tool to measure cost-effectiveness is currently impeding the fuller development of a preventative strategy and this clearly requires major attention. Yet, enhancing the quality of life of older people is not only a valid end in itself but can help them maintain the ability and motivation to care for themselves. Quality of life may not easily lend itself to measurements of cost-effectiveness but if the meaning of 'best value' is to be judged in terms which extend beyond short-term financial exigencies, then the value older people accord low level preventative services cannot be ignored.

The challenge for policy makers at local and national levels remains to look beyond short-term demands and the boundaries of what they perceive as important, and to take on board what older people themselves value in terms of maintaining their independence:

> "I prefer to be in my own home and, you know, look after myself as much as I possibly can *with* that bit of help."

References

Anchor (1996) *Preventative services for older people and community care: Findings from a joint policy seminar,* Oxford: Anchor Trust.

Arber, S. and Ginn, J. (1991) *Gender and later life: A sociological analysis of resources and constraints,* London: Sage.

Audit Commission (1997) *The coming of age: Improving care services for older people,* London: Audit Commission.

Boateng, P. (1997) Address to the Health and Social Care Conference, Gatwick, 2 December.

Bowling, A., Grundy, E. and Farquhar, M. (1997) *Living well into old age,* Social Care Research Findings 95, York: Joseph Rowntree Foundation.

Caldock, K. and Wenger, G.C. (1992) 'Health and social service provision for elderly people: the need for a rural model', in A. Gilg (ed) *Progress in rural policy and planning: Volume 2,* London: Belhaven Press.

DoH (Department of Health) (1989) *Caring for people: Community care in the next decade and beyond,* Cm 849, London, HMSO.

DoH (1990) *Community care in the next decade and beyond: Policy guidance,* London: HMSO.

DoH (1997) *The new NHS – Modern, dependable,* London: The Stationary Office.

DoH (1998) *Our healthier nation: A contract for health,* Cm 3854, London: The Stationary Office.

Gray, M. (1988) 'Living environments for the elderly. 1: Living at home', in N. Wells and C. Freer (eds) *The ageing population: Burden or challenge?,* Basingstoke: Macmillan.

Gurney, C. and Means, R. (1993) 'The meaning of home in later life', in S. Arber and M. Evandrou (eds) *Ageing, independence and the life course,* London: Jessica Kingsley.

Henwood, M. (1992) *Through a glass darkly: Community care and elderly people,* London: King's Fund Institute.

Henwood, M., Lewis, H. and Waddington, E. (1998) 'I'll tell you what I want', *Community Care,* 22-28 January, pp 28-9.

House of Commons Health Committee (1996) *Long-term care: Future provision and funding,* Session 1995-96, Third Report HC59-1, London: HMSO.

Hughes, B. (1990) 'Quality of life', in S. Peace (ed) *Researching social gerontology,* London: Sage.

Langan, J., Means, R. and Rolfe, S. (1996) *Maintaining independence in later life: Older people speaking,* Oxford: Anchor Trust.

Morris, J. (1993) *Independent lives? Community care and disabled people,* Basingstoke: Macmillan.

Oakley, A. (1974) *The sociology of housework,* London: Martin Robertson.

Sidell, M. (1995) *Health in old age,* Buckingham: Open University Press.

Sinclair, I. and Williams, J. (1990a) 'Elderly people: coping and quality of life', in I. Sinclair, R. Parker, D. Leat and J. Williams (eds) *The kaleidoscope of care: A review of research on welfare provision for elderly people,* London: HMSO.

Sinclair, I. and Williams, J. (1990b) 'Domiciliary services', in I. Sinclair, R. Parker, D. Leat and J. Williams (eds) *The kaleidoscope of care: A review of research on welfare provision for elderly people,* London: HMSO.

Sixsmith, A. (1986) 'Independence and home in later life', in D. Phillipson, M. Bernard and P. Strang (eds) *Dependency and interdependency in old age: Theoretical perspectives and policy alternatives,* London: Croom Helm.

SSI (Social Services Inspectorate) (1987) *From home help to home care: An analysis of policy resourcing and service management,* London: DHSS.

Stevenson, O. (1989) *Age and vulnerability: A guide to better care,* London: Edward Arnold.

Tinker, A. (1996) *Older people in modern society,* London: Longman.

Warnes, A.M. (1993) *'Being old: old people and the burdens of burden',* Ageing and Society, vol 13, pp 297-338.

Wenger, G.C. (1992) *Help in old age – Facing up to change,* Liverpool: Liverpool University Press.

Willcocks, D., Peace, S. and Kellaher, L. (1987) *Private lives in public places: A research-based critique of residential life in local authority old people's homes,* London: Tavistock.

Wistow, G. (1997) *Policy and political comment in prevention works,* Oxford: Anchor Trust.

Wistow, G. and Lewis, H. (1997) *Preventative services for older people: Current approaches and future opportunities,* Oxford: Anchor Trust.